ARYUVEDIC MEDICINE FOR WESTERNERS

Jim Elliott

Contents

INTRODUCTION

This little book is something I never thought I would write. Until recently I had no idea of Aryuvedic Medicines until a friend of mine became ill and his sister – a conventional doctor – suggested using Aryuvedic medicine. I thought this was only because they were from India. So, I went along with them and was quite stunned at the difference.

When I collected him from the hospital, I was given a given a carrier bag with 16 different drugs and it became a daily ritual sorting these out.

I scanned and sent the drug list to my friend's sister and pointed out that there was no real improvement in his condition. He was weak, easily tired, and generally not himself.

I received two Aryuvedic medicines through the post and gave them to him on the basis that the worst they could do was nothing.

I was so wrong. Within 10 days he was considerably better, and his doctor started cutting down on the medicines.

Now several months later we are down to 3 – and they are reducing.

So that started my interest. Well, I thought, if it was over 3,000 years old they must know something.

I have since pointed people in this route and have seen some surprising results. I would add that I am not a healthcare professional, so I always tell people to check first.

I hope this little book – which is not meant to be an academic reference or explanation – will help you discover a fascinating and effective method.

A QUICK OVERVIEW OF THE CONCEPTS OF ARUYVEDIC MEDICINE.

ORIGINS AND EVOLUTION OF AYURVEDA

Our journey into the world of Ayurveda begins thousands of years ago. Let's bend time and space a little and travel to ancient India, where the roots of Ayurveda run deep. In the dawn of civilization, when mankind was still learning to conquer fire, the learned sages of ancient India were busy developing a complete system of medicine, based on the profound understanding of the universe and its relation to human anatomy.

THE VEDIC ERA AND ITS HEALTH PRACTICES

A time when scriptures were enlightened whispers passed down from guru to disciple, and ancient texts were the epitome of wisdom, the Vedic era forms the milieu wherein Ayurveda was born. Rooted in the Vedas, specifically in the Atharvaveda, Ayurveda emerged as an integral part of the spiritual and philosophical dialogue that engaged these wise early humans. It was not merely a doctrine of medical treatment but a lifestyle manual, instructing ways to maintain health and lead a balanced life.

HISTORICAL DEVELOPMENT OF AYURVEDA

From the teachings of the Vedas, distinctive texts dedicated to Ayurveda began to take shape. The celebrated "Charaka Samhita" and "Sushruta Samhita," along with various other treatises, marked significant milestones in the evolution of Ayurveda. These compendiums meticulously broke down every aspect of health, wellness, and disease treatment. They spoke of the principles that govern our biology - the Doshas, the art of healing surgery, how every life form had a spirit, and most importantly about Ayurveda as the science of life that encompassed the body, mind, and spirit.

Deeply influenced by the philosophies of Sankhya and Vaisheshika, Ayurveda emphasizes the interconnectedness of the mind, body, and spirit. The concept of 'Purusha' symbolizes consciousness, the subtle energies that comprise our being, while 'Prakruti' stands for matter, including our physical bodies. The balance between these entities, their interaction and reactions, forms the base of Ayurveda.

Through this book, we will further decode these concepts, trying to understand our ancient sages' wisdom in bringing forth an all-inclusive, holistic therapeutic practice like Ayurveda.

THE PRINCIPLES OF AYURVEDA

With the essence of the ancient wisdom assimilated, now we venture deeper on our quest to understanding Ayurveda. Let's delve into the core principles that form the backbone of this age-old healthcare system.

THE FIVE ELEMENTAL THEORY

In the heart of Ayurvedic philosophy lies the five-elemental theory. These elements- space (Akasha), air (Vayu), fire (Agni), water (Jala), and earth (Prithvi)- are not just physical entities; they represent different characteristics that are observed in nature and within our bodies. Let's imagine a roaring campfire. The heat and flames represent 'fire,' the smoke symbolizes 'air,' the space it reaches represents 'space'; the residual ashes symbolize 'earth,' and the moisture in the ashes reflects 'water.' Understand that every physical composition in the universe is a unique, intricate blend of these five elements, including our bodies.

DOSHA THEORY - VATA, PITTA, KAPHA

You might be wondering, how do these elements manifest in our bodies? This is where 'Doshas' enter the conversation. Doshas are functional energies within us, formed by the combination of two elements. There are three Doshas- Vata (space and air), Pitta (fire and water), and Kapha (water and earth). These Doshas influence our physical, mental, and emotional tendencies. As unique as a thumbprint, everyone has an individual combination of these doshas, which is predetermined at the moment of conception.

AYURVEDA, BALANCE AND THE ART OF HEALTHY LIVING

As we delve deeper into the Ayurvedic doctrine, we move away from the theoretical and embark on the practical aspects of this age-old wisdom. Here, we discover the art of balance that Ayurveda imparts to us, leading to a healthy, fulfilling life.

THE SCIENCE OF BALANCE

In Ayurveda, health is considered as a delicate equilibrium of the body, mind, and spirit. This equilibrium is maintained by the Doshas – Vata, Pitta, and Kapha. Each having a unique blend of these doshas, which is established at birth and remains constant throughout life. But our environment, dietary choices, seasons, lifestyle, and mental-emotional states cause these Doshas to fluctuate, leading to imbalances. Ayurveda provides us with a roadmap to understand these changes and how to return to our balanced state.

THE THREE PILLARS OF HEALTH

Often referred to as the three pillars of life, Ahara (diet), Nidra (sleep), and Brahmacharya (regulated sexual activity) are three essential factors in maintaining health according to Ayurveda. Eating a diet that's appropriate for our 'Prakriti', getting adequate sleep, and maintaining a healthy sexual life, form the bedrock of a balanced life. We will investigate these pillars further, considering how they function holistically to support a physically resilient and mentally vibrant existence.

Conceptualizing a balanced routine, Ayurveda also suggests a lifestyle regimen, called Dinacharya. This comprises a set of self-care practices that need to be performed daily, starting from the point of waking up till going back to sleep. The unique aspect of these practices is their consideration for the daily cycles of nature, such as the rise and fall of the sun and changes in climatic conditions. We'll explore Dinacharya in great depth, outlining how the timely performance of these practices keeps us aligned with nature, helping to sustain optimum health.

We believe that Ayurveda, at its core, is a way of life. It empowers us with knowledge about our unique constitutions, enabling us to navigate our lives towards balance and health. Together, as we continue to journey through the ayurvedic odyssey, we will unravel more of its wisdom, which will hopefully bring about a holistic transformation in the way we live and perceive health.

THE AYURVEDIC APPROACH TO NUTRITION

As we journey further, we arrive at one of the most impactful aspects of Ayurveda - Nutrition. The ancient sages deeply understood that the food we consume serves not just as mere fuel, but as the primal source of nourishment, replenishment, and healing.

FOOD – THE MOST POTENT MEDICINE

Ayurveda teaches us that we are essentially what we digest., a premise that echoes the modern understanding of our gut being our "second brain." Every morsel we eat influences our 'Doshic balance,' and hence our health. It advocates a Sattvic diet that is fresh, nutritious, tasty, and suitable for one's unique constitution. This chapter uncovers the potential of food as medicine and the importance of mindful eating.

THE SIX TASTES & THEIR SIGNIFICANCE

Ayurveda recognizes six tastes: sweet, sour, salty, bitter, pungent and astringent. Each taste corresponds to the elemental composition and holds a different effect on the Doshas. Ayurvedic nutrition emphasizes including all six tastes in our meals to ensure a balanced diet. The intricate understanding of how each taste affects our body forms the crux of Ayurvedic nutritional advice.

AGNI – THE DIGESTIVE FIRE

The importance of what we eat is well understood, however, Ayurveda underlines one other factor of equal importance - how well we are able to digest the food. Agni, the digestive fire, determines this. A balanced Agni ensures optimum digestion and absorption of nutrients while warding off the formation of Ama, which is undigested food residue leading to disease.

By understanding and applying these principles, Ayurveda helps us create a healthier relationship with our food. But the journey doesn't end here. The next chapter unveils deeper dimensions of Ayurvedic wisdom. We still have many more fascinating aspects to unfold, leading not just to a healthier existence, but a blissful life experience.

AYURVEDA AND THE MIND-BODY CONNECTION

As we delve further into our exploration, we introduce a core principle of Ayurveda that has revolutionized modern medicine: the mind-body connection. For Ayurveda, the seamless dialogue between the body and mind is central to achieving optimal health.

THE DANCE OF THE BODY AND MIND

Ayurvedic wisdom underscores the inseparable bond between body, mind, and consciousness. Its teachings remind us that emotions profoundly influence our physical health as our bodies echo our mental and emotional states in the form of physiological responses. Likewise, a healthy, nourished body creates a fertile ground for a resilient mind.

TAMING THE MIND

Ayurveda advances certain mental disciplines in maintaining a balanced mind-body connection. Key among these are the practice of mindfulness and meditation. These practices ensure a calm, focused mind, free from the agitation contributed by the chaos of day-to-day living. By shaping and disciplining our minds, we can carve a path to overall well-being and harmony.

EMOTIONAL WELL-BEING

In Ayurveda, maintaining a balance amongst the Doshas extends to mental health as well. Practices such as self-reflection, positive affirmations, and cultivating constructive emotional characteristics form an integral part of fostering emotional wellness. By adopting these practices, we can undo the habitual patterns that disrupt our mental and physical health and lead us to a state of inner freedom.

Our intrepid journey through Ayurvedic wisdom continues to unfurl, affirming that it isn't just an alternative health system, but a way of life that reverberates with vitality. As we continue this exploration into Ayurveda's profound knowledge, we inch closer to comprehending the unity of body, mind, and spirit, illuminating the path to enriched health and happiness.

INTERLACING YOGA AND AYURVEDA

Ah, now we venture into a domain where the riveting sister sciences of Yoga and Ayurveda beautifully intertwine. You see, Ayurveda, the science of life, and Yoga, the science of union, are deeply interconnected, complementing each other magnificently.

THE SCIENCE OF UNION - YOGA

Yoga, much more than just a physical exercise, is a profound spiritual path focused on unifying the body, mind, and spirit. The ultimate aim of Yoga is to attain Samadhi, a state of transcendent consciousness where the individual self-dissolves into the universal.

AYURVEDA AND YOGA – THE PERFECT AMALGAMATION

Ayurveda and Yoga are two sides of the same coin, never complete without each other. Just as Ayurveda advises particular diets and lifestyles for different Dosha types, it similarly suggests specific yoga asanas. The forms of yoga, pranayama, and meditation can be tailored to an individual's Dosha, thus ensuring optimal health and balance.

Yoga provides us with the method to regulate life energy or Prana. Ayurveda, upfront about the significance of Prana, considers its imbalance as the root of all sickness. Here, we comprehend how Pranayama, the yogic practice of breath control, fits into the Ayurvedic perspective, aiding in harmonizing Prana and bringing vitality and vibrancy to our being.

As we gradually thread through the profundity of these sister sciences, we come to realize that the balance and health we hope to achieve are not distant dreams, but something well within our reach--in the end, we are the artisans of our body and psyche.

Our journey doesn't conclude here, however. As we proceed through the world of Ayurveda and Yoga, more revelations await us. Stay tuned, the journey has just begun.

THE AYURVEDIC KITCHEN – WHERE FOOD BECOMES MEDICINE

Leaping ahead, we unlock the doors to the Ayurvedic Kitchen, where food transforms into the best form of medicine. Ayurveda's intricate understanding of nutrition and digestion pivots on the notion that food has a dynamic impact on our physical and mental well-being.

THE IMPORTANCE OF 'AGNI'

Essential to understanding Ayurvedic nutrition is the concept of 'Agni' or digestive fire. This ingenious metaphorical fire within us digests our food, generating energy while discarding toxins. Picture Agni as your internal wellbeing manager, looking over health, vitality, and longevity.

THE SIX TASTES OF NUTRITION

Venture into the diverse world of Ayurvedic flavours, all six of them, each having a unique influence on our Doshas. Sweet, sour, salty, bitter, astringent, and pungent - there's a delicacy and art to combining these tastes to create balanced, nourishing meals that feed not only our bodies but our spirits too.

FOOD FOR YOUR DOSHA

Navigating the nutritional landscape isn't about riding a wave of fad diets. Instead, Ayurveda guides us towards foods that best suit our individual constitution or Dosha. Aligning your meals to pacify your prominent Dosha can contribute significantly to maintaining equilibrium and warding off disease.

Meandering through this vast Ayurvedic culinary landscape opens up new avenues of understanding food, not just as a source of sustenance but a profound healing agent. As we progress further, you'll find how every morsel you ingest and the way you consume it can profoundly impact your overall health and vitality. So stay curious, my comrade, the journey is just as important as the destination.

THE AYURVEDIC PATH TO WELLNESS

Now, let us journey down the road of holistic well-being, where the tempos of Ayurveda furnish an age-old path to wellness. The melodic cadence of holistic health care teaches that invincible health and well-being cannot be unlocked through physical care alone; we must tend to our emotional and spiritual domains too.

AYURVEDA'S MULTIDIMENSIONAL APPROACH

Any disruption that appears on the body's surface stems from deeper layers of consciousness. Isn't that intriguing? The Ayurvedic approach isn't confined to treating the symptoms but primarily aims to eliminate the root cause, aligning body, mind, and spirit to its natural state of harmony.

NATURE'S PHARMACY – AYURVEDIC HERBS

From the roots of the earth emerge nature's pharmacy, where thousands of herbs dance with medicinal properties. Each herb, with its unique healing power, unfolds the potential to rebalance our Doshas and spark innate healing drifts. Dare to navigate our diverse herbal terrain, and you shall discover natures' many miracles.

HEALING ROUTINES – DINACHARYA AND RITUCHARYA

And herein we sow the seeds of habit, for Ayurveda portends that a well-regimented daily routine, or Dinacharya, can significantly help maintain good health. Alongside, the observance of seasonal routines, Ritucharya, ensures that our bodies synchronise with nature's rhythm, shielding us against seasonal fluctuations and ailments.

We dare to dream of a world where each being can access the profound wisdom of Ayurveda to nurture their wellbeing.

As we culminate this chapter, we leave with the thought that this ancient science of life offers an umbrella of wellness. It teaches us that everything we need for health and happiness lies within us. Stay with us as there's still much to explore.

A LITTLE MORE DETAIL OF THE KEY CONCEPTS

A FULLER DELVING INTO THE DOSHAS

Out here in the universes' grand expanse, we encounter energy in all its forms - the scorching sun, the soft breeze, the tranquil sea, the towering mountains. Love it or despise it, energy keeps the world's wheel spinning.

A similar energy vibrates within us, divided into three essential categories or Doshas – Vata, Pitta, and Kapha. Imagine them as invisible life forces, the cosmos' conductors silently orchestrating the symphony of life within our bodies.

Let's tune into the rhythms of the Doshas and decode their mysterious melodies. Get ready to dive headfirst into the enchanting whirlpool of Ayurvedic theory!

VATA - THE WIND ENERGY

Imagine Vata as the wind, ever so swift and free, carrying movements within our bodies. Anything that moves, twists, circulates, or flows sashays to Vata's tune. This beloved maestro claims dominion over the nervous system and governs all motion, including blood flow, elimination of wastes, breathing, and the movement of thoughts across our minds. Yep, that's right; your thoughts are also under Vata's command.

You're quite possibly in the Vata gang if you have a lean body and move faster than Usain Bolt at the buffet table. Born under Vata's star, you're a jet-setter, constantly on the move, zipping from this to that with boundless energy. However, when Vata fluctuates, it's synonymous with a tremendous thunderstorm. The calm seas become turbulent with anxiety, fear, and an overactive mind. Fret not, mates, with grounding foods, a warm and cozy environment, and a structured routine, Vata remains in friendly harmony.

PITTA - THE FIRE ENERGY

Next up, ladies and gentlemen, raise your glasses to Pitta, the fire energy. Burning strong and bright, Pitta lights up digestion and metabolism. Anything you digest, food, water, experiences, or emotions, stokes Pitta's flame.

You can easily pick out someone dominated by Pitta; they're fiery, passionate, and focused. A Pitta-charged person is blessed with a radiant complexion and medium build. They are razor-sharp and possess a competitive spirit. No mystery remains unsolved in the hands of a Pitta detective.

But, when the Pitta thermometer rises too high, be prepared for volcanic eruptions! An overbearing Pitta generation can lead to anger, jealousy, inflammation, and a thunder-like ego! The golden rule to pacify Pitta's antagonism is simple: stay cool, and not just in demeanour. Cool foods, surroundings, and temperaments serve to soothe the feisty, fiery Pitta.

KAPHA - THE EARTH AND WATER ENERGY

Finally, meet Kapha, the earth and water energy. Visualize Kapha as the reassuring forest floor or the calm unperturbed lake, firm and tranquil. Kapha's mission is to provide structure, stability, and lubrication for our bodies. It's the glue holding our bones, muscles, and tendons together, and it's this moisture that keeps our skin dewy.

If you're blessed with robust health, a sturdy build, and a calming presence, you're a natural charmer in Kapha's club. People with a Kapha constitution are the human embodiment of zen, calm as a summer's breeze, patient, loyal, and enduring. Now, when Kapha's harmony falters, it can make you feel heavy, lethargic, clingy, and resistant to change, mimicking a stuck wooden wheel. The key to maintaining Kapha's equilibrium is stimulation. Frequent exercise, new experiences, variety in diet, all help to keep Kapha's energy vibrant and mobile.

There you have it, the grand orchestra of Doshas in subtle harmony. Remember, we're not married to only one Dosha but are all a unique mix of these vital energies.

The Doshas shape not just our physical attributes, but our emotional and mental characteristics too, creating the music to the grand opera of our lives.

So, the next time you find yourself out of tune, look no further. Sync with your Doshas and sway to their rhythm, and you'll soon find yourself back on life's harmonious track!

MATTERS DIGESTIVE

Ladies and gentlemen, let's switch on the spotlight and guide its beam onto our entertainment for the evening. Meet, Agni and Ama, arguably Ayurveda's yin and yang, two sides of the same coin, our body's indispensable secret agents. They are diametrically opposite stand on health and wellness but are powerfully intertwined in a mesmerizing tango.

AGRABATTI TO AGNI - THE DIGESTIVE FIRE

First on stage is the heartthrob of wellbeing, Agni, Ayurveda's Digestive Fire, our in-house celebrity tucked away in the belly. Our physical health, emotional stability, and strength of immunity are all fiery fans of Agni.

"When Agni is in a balanced state, an individual will remain healthy, free from disorders. But, if Agni becomes impaired, the digestion process is affected leading to the production of Ama and eventually disease." - Charaka Samhita.

Can you feel the warmth radiating from Agni already? This essence of fire is your best friend, despite the hot temperament, for it holds power over the transformation. How we digest food, how our cells metabolize nutrients, even our ability to process emotions and thoughts - all dance to the tunes of fiery Agni.

Now, let's zip down to our gut microcosm. See that golden pyre of Agni blazing gloriously? This fire breaks down the food we consume into the simplest forms for our body to absorb. When Agni rages at its optimal, every morsel you eat is transformed into nourishment. Your body hums with vitality, your thoughts are sharp, and emotions are stable.

On the flip side, if Agni's flame dwindles, it struggles to metabolize food efficiently. There's insufficient heat, and rather than being converted into nourishment, the food transforms into toxic sludge, the infamous AMA.

A MOVIE MOMENT WITH AMA - THE TOXIC SLUDGE

Enter Ama, the villain of our wellbeing saga, the toxic residue that results from incomplete digestion. Portrayed as the root cause of all diseases in Ayurveda's grand narrative, Ama is the by-product of imbalanced Agni, the Jekyll to its Hyde.

An individual with an accumulation of Ama experiences a plethora of symptoms. Ever felt heavy, bloated, experience fatigue or cloudy thinking? You've had a meet-and-greet with Ama.

Ama is at heart an intruder, an uninvited guest who crashed the health party. It was allowed entry by sub-optimum Agni, and now it sloths around, seeping into various nooks and crannies, gumming up the works. Depending upon where it accumulates, Ama colours the symptoms.

However, our villain Ama isn't invincible; it faces destruction once our blazing hero Agni gains strength.

AGNI & AMA: AN AYURVEDIC ADVENTURE

In the Ayurvedic narrative, the main characters, Agni and Ama, enormously impact our health and lifestyle.

Agni, our hero, an essential cornerstone of our digestive system, needs to burn bright and steady to ensure efficient digestion and absorption of food. Its inexplicable energy fuels our essence and keeps us vibrant and healthy.

If ever Agni's flame weakens, the villain Ama seizes an opportunity to overrun our bodies, leading to imbalance, illness and disease.

In the grand stage of life, the gut is a central character. When the transformative fire, Agni, is balanced, and the toxic villain Ama is minimized, the gut thrives, paving the path to overall health and wellbeing.

The understanding of Agni and Ama reveals one truth - health is rooted in powerful digestion. It erodes Ayurveda's profound wisdom nugget - we aren't just what we eat, but what we digest.

Through warm, cooked, and easy-to-digest foods, right eating practices, and a balanced lifestyle, Agni thrives, keeping villainous Ama out of the scene.

There you have it, all the tantalizing drama our bodies host daily with Agni and Ama. Embark on the riveting journey of exploring your own body's unique Agni, with its constant affair with Ama, and you'll steer your health towards the gate of true wellbeing.

Stay strong, keep the fire burning, and remember - health imbalances may seem vexing but come with illuminating insights, spoonful of self-reflections, and dollops of wisdom.

Keep the fire of curiosity alive, and let's continue the journey into the magical realms of Ayurveda!

PANCHAKARM – ARYUVEDIC DETOX

Ever thought of hitting the reset button on your body's health? Taking that much-needed vacation from the daily hustle? Welcome on board to the blissful journey of Panchakarma, 'The Five Actions,' your ultimate detox vacation. Let's travel through a relaxing, rejuvenating, and radical transformation.

DISCOVERY OF PANCHAKARM

Pancha-what? Featuring front and centre in the timeless saga of Ayurveda, Panchakarma is a series of treatments designed to detoxify and rejuvenate the body. Modern lifestyles sum up to be a carnival of toxins, stress, unhealthy eating, and sedentary routines. Enter Panchakarma, the star of Ayurveda, countering the demanding rigors of life and restoring us to vitality.

THE BENEVOLENT PANCHAKARMA

Think of Panchakarma as your health's personal SWAT team sent to remove the toxic build-up (Ama) from your body, resetting your Agni (digestive fire). What follows is better digestion, a robust immune system, and a vibrant glow surpassing any Instagram filter.

Apart from its detoxifying effects, Panchakarma paves the way for deep relaxation, mental clarity, and emotional healing. Panchakarma, hence, is more than a mere spa-like indulgence; it's a pathway to profound self-transformation.

NAVIGATING THROUGH THE FIVE ACTIONS

Panchakarma, true to its name, incorporates five key actions; Vamana, Virechana, Basti, Nasya, and Raktamokshana.

- Vamana (Therapeutic Vomiting): Far from being a bad memory of a nasty flu, Vamana is a closely supervised procedure to expel excess Kapha from the body.

- Virechana(Therapeutic Purgation): Another 'not-at-a-dinner-party topic', Virechana helps eliminate excess Pitta toxins from the body.

- Basti(Enema Therapy): Hold on to your hats folks! Ayurvedic enemas come in two variants - herbal oil enemas (Anuvasana) and herbal decoction enemas (Asthhapana/Niruha).

- Nasya (Nasal administration): Get this, health through the nostrils! Instilling medicated oil through the nostrils purges accumulated Kapha toxins from the neck and head.

- Raktamokshana(Blood Letting): The most rarely used treatment, it's a blood purification process and remedial measure for disorders caused by vitiated blood.

TAKING OFF WITH PANCHAKARMA

Dive into the Panchakarma adventure with Purvakarma, the pre-procedure practices. This stage prepares your body, like an aircraft gaining the necessary momentum before take-off.

In Ayurveda, we have two significant flying companions – Snehana (Oleation) and Swedana (Sweating). Snehana involves internal and external oiling of the body, and Swedana is a luxurious herbal steam therapy.

Together, these dynamic duos awaken the dormant toxins, softening and dislodging them from tissues. Like coaxing children out of a candy store, they move these toxins towards the gastrointestinal tract, ready for elimination.

LANDING WITH PASCHATKARMA

Completing your Panchakarma voyage is the Paschatkarma, a series of regimens to restore balance post-therapy, like adjusting to ground reality after an exhilarating flight. Your practitioner may suggest a specialized diet, Ayurvedic medicines or herbs, lifestyle modifications, or yoga and meditation.

THE PANCHAKARMA TRANSFORMATION

Panchakarma is a personalized Ayurvedic retreat, each individual experiencing it differently, like the varying hues of a soulful sunset. The detox process can sometimes stir up emotions, offering windows to profound personal insight. Among its tangible souvenirs are glowing complexion, restored strength, increased mental clarity, improved digestion, and a sudden surge in friend requests from intestines to neurons, praising your flawless life choices.

The Panchakarma experience might sound intense, like a bizarre detox carnival where you're both the audience and performer. Yet, it's your unique pathway to a rejuvenated version of you. Witness bodies sigh relief, spirits dance joyfully, and revel in the luxurious purification offered by Panchakarma.

Embark on the beautiful journey back to health and harmony. Flip through the pages of self-discovery, sift through layers of mind-body connection, and dip in the healing springs of Panchakarma.

This fascinating Ayurvedic detox is more than just a health regimen; it's a doorway to reconnect with your innermost self, dancing to the rhythm of nourished health, radiant glow, and infinite vitality. Bon voyage, health enthusiasts!

ARYUVEDIC AND WESTERN MEDICINE

Welcome, enlightened seekers, to the fascinating intersection of ancient wisdom and modern science. This exhilarating narrative unfolds at the crossroads of Ayurveda, the age-old science of life, and Western Medicine, the empirically driven modern healthcare system. Buckle up and enjoy the ride through this harmonious integration and the exciting prospects of scientific research.

A TALE OF TWO MEDICINES

When unveiling the curtain of Ayurveda and Western medicine, we uncover two spectacularly different healing arts. Ayurveda, with its roots deeply embedded in the Indian subcontinent, is a holistic healing science focusing on the individual's mind, body, and spirit.

In contrast, Western Medicine, born out of the Scientific Revolution, operates on evidence-based paradigms, emphasizing physical symptoms and disease treatment.

WISDOM MEETS SCIENCE: A GENTLE EMBRACE

In an age where optimal health is the supreme quest, integrating Ayurveda with Western Medicine seems like a match made in medical heaven.

This holistic union draws upon Ayurveda's preventive and lifestyle-based approach and Western medicine's strength in acute care and cutting-edge technology. It's like bringing together an experienced grandmaster and a whip-smart whiz kid for an exciting, new health venture.

THE POWER OF PREVENTION AND PERSONALIZATION

Ayurveda brings to the table its invaluable understanding of the individual 'Prakriti' (constitution) and 'Dosha' (biological energies) balance. Imagine your health like a personalized piece of playlist tailored precisely to your unique rhythm and beats. Recognizing individual differences, Ayurveda weaves a custom-made regimen of diet, lifestyle and herbal supplements to maintain balance, thus preventing diseases.

Western medicine, traditionally designed with a 'one-size-fits-all' approach, starts to embrace the Ayurvedic perspective of individual uniqueness. This marriage of preventative care with the technologically advanced diagnosis and treatment opens up possibilities for truly personalized medicine.

IMPLEMENTING INTEGRATIVE MEDICINE: CHALLENGES AND REWARDS

How do we create an integrative healthcare landscape combining Ayurveda's millennia-old wisdom with the strengths of Western medicine? It's no easy feat, for sure. The challenge lies in standardizing Ayurvedic practices by Western scientific criteria, wrestling through regulatory issues, and bridging cultural understandings.

Yet, the reward of integrative medicine is worth embarking on this transformative journey. It builds a healthcare approach that is proactive rather than reactive, preventive rather than curative, and individual-based rather than generalized.

SCIENTIFIC RESEARCH: THE BRIDGE CONNECTING AYURVEDA AND WESTERN MEDICINE

The path to integration shines brightly with the beacon of scientific research. Herbal pharmacology is one research area where Ayurveda and Western medicine intersect seamlessly.

Turmeric, a common Indian household spice, is a stand-out star in scientific research. It's a high-five moment when Western medical research validates Ayurveda's claims on Turmeric's anti-inflammatory, antioxidant, and anti-cancer properties.

THE STAGE OF EMPIRICAL EVIDENCE

To strengthen the structure of integrative medicine, more Ayurvedic concepts, methodologies, and therapies require quantifiable validation through Western research models.

With evidence-based studies, we bridge the gap of understanding between the two systems. When peer-reviewed studies back the Ayurvedic practices, it lends credibility and facilitates acceptance among Western practitioners.

NAVIGATING THE JOURNEY TOWARDS INTEGRATIVE HEALTHCARE

We stand at an exciting crossroads on our health journey. Merging Ayurveda's preventative and personalized approach with Western medicine's technological advancements can pave a new, holistic terrain in healthcare.

The thriving integration of Ayurveda and Western medicine isn't just an amalgamation of two distinct philosophies. It's the weaving of a new narrative that pulls the threads from each, creating a tapestry of health and wellness that exhibits the richness, depth, and synergy of both.

As we navigate through this transdisciplinary fusion, let's marvel at the wisdom of adopting past's knowledge into present's advancement to cultivate a healthier future.

Embrace the complementary strengths of the ancient Ayurveda and modern Western medicine and remember - the ultimate winner in this integrative journey is you, the seeker of optimal health and wellbeing!

IMPROVING DIGESTION WITH ARYUVEDA

Welcome to the realm of Ayurveda and the intriguing pathway to holistically high-powered digestion. Let's embark on a journey that meanders through the realm of Ayurveda, offering golden nuggets of wisdom to help spruce up your digestive health.

AYURVEDA AND AGNI: THE FIERY DUO

Let's turn the spotlight on 'Agni,' the sacred digestive fire in Ayurvedic philosophy. It's not just about breaking down the food physically, but also about assimilating nutrients and eliminating waste efficiently. The Agni's strength steers the ship of physical health, mental clarity, and overall vitality. Sounds like a fiery superhero of digestion, doesn't it?

KEY PILLARS FOR POWERING UP DIGESTION

A durable digestive foundation rests on three essential pillars: how you eat, what you eat, and when you eat. Remember, Ayurveda doesn't deal with 'one-size-fits-all.' So, these pillars will vary based on your unique constitution or 'Dosha' (Vata, Pitta, and Kapha).

'HOW' TO EAT: THE MINDFUL MUNCH

Ayurveda emphasizes the experience of eating. The first cardinal rule—eat mindfully. Marvel at the colours on your plate, take in the aroma, chew thoroughly, and savour every bite. Be fully present in the moment with no laptops, phones, or books as dining partners. This practice dramatically increases digestion and absorption, ensuring you reap the full benefits of your meals.

'WHAT' TO EAT: THE BALANCE BETWEEN TASTY AND HEALTHY

The second pillar—pay careful attention to what lands on your plate. The Ayurvedic diet revolves around the concept of six tastes—sweet, sour, salty, bitter, pungent, and astringent. As much as the palette permits, include all six tastes in your meals. It promotes balance, satiety, and a diverse intake of nutrients.

Also, prefer freshly cooked, warm, and organic food over processed or packaged foods. Fresh fruit, vegetables, whole grains, and lean protein sources are the stars of the Ayurvedic diet.

'WHEN' TO EAT: THE CLOCK OF FOOD

The 'when' of eating is just as crucial in Ayurveda. Have your largest meal at midday when the sun is high, and digestive fire, Agni, is at its strongest. Indeed, not a fan of late-night snacks or meals, Ayurveda prefers lighter dinners eaten a few hours before bed. Align your meals with nature's rhythms, and the digestive tune is set!

SPICE UP YOUR LIFE

Spices are Ayurveda's secret for stoking the digestive fire. A variety of spices like cumin, ginger, fennel, turmeric, and black pepper can be your kitchen warriors, fighting bloating, gas, and indigestion. These spices are not only flavourful but also ignite digestion, aid absorption, and eliminate waste.

AYURVEDIC SUPERHEROES OF DIGESTION: HERBS AND REMEDIES

Ayurveda appreciates and utilizes nature's pharmacy. Aloe Vera supports healthy elimination, Triphala aids in detoxification, and Liquorice soothes the stomach lining. But remember, always consult an Ayurvedic practitioner before starting any herbal supplement.

ABHYANGA: A WARM EMBRACE OF OIL

Keen to muster up some more Ayurvedic magic? Say hello to Abhyanga, a self-massage using warm oil. It stimulates the digestive organs, reduces stress, and promotes overall wellbeing.

END OF THE DAY VICTORY: A SOUND SLEEP

Never underestimate the power of a good night's sleep. A sound sleep gives your digestive system the much-needed downtime to repair and rejuvenate. While late-night munchies and gadgets are the enemies of sleep, sticking to a regular sleep schedule and a calming bedtime routine can take you a long way on the road to restful slumber.

And there you have it—a gentle nudge toward reimagining digestion the Ayurvedic way. Remember, embarking on the Ayurvedic journey is like tuning the strings of your digestive guitar to the rhythm of nature.

The beauty of Ayurveda lies not in a hurried pursuit of quick fixes but a more profound awareness and alignment with one's unique rhythms.

So, get ready to stoke your Agni, indulge in mindful munching, become friends with spices- the delightful digestive warriors, and greet the sun, nature's best alarm clock! Enjoy the food rainbow and fall in love with your digestion all over again. After all, as we say in Ayurveda, 'you are what you digest.' Happy Digesting!

SOME IMPORTANT TIME-HONOURED ARYUVEDIC MEDICINES

Now let's delve into the world of thirty significant Ayurvedic constituents and their applications. Buckle up for this exciting exploration of nature's pharmacy:

Ashwagandha (Winter Cherry)

An adaptogenic herb supreme for mitigating anxiety and insomnia. Primary constituents - Withanolides, Withaferins.

Brahmi (Waterhyssop)

A brain-boosting wonder improving memory and cognition. Components include Bacosides.

Long Pepper (Pippali)

An esteemed remedy for the respiratory and digestive system. Active constituents include Piperine and Piperlongumine.

Triphala

A remarkable trio of Amalaki (Indian Gooseberry), Bibhitaki (Beleric), and Haritaki (Black Myrobalan), playing the role of a gentle bowel cleanser.

Chyawanprash

A health-intensifying supplement nurturing overall wellness, primarily composed of Amla (Indian Gooseberry) and numerous other herbal ingredients.

Arjuna

Nature's heart ally, favouring cardiovascular wellbeing. It's rich in multiple flavonoids and tannins.

Neem (Indian Lilac)

Skin's best friend due to its purifying properties. The key players are Azadirachtin and Nimbin.

Shatavari (Wild Asparagus)

A rejuvenate herb promoting female health and fertility, containing steroidal saponins.

Tulsi (Holy Basil)

An incredible immunity booster addressing common colds and respiratory conditions. Eugenol is the primary compound here.

Guggul (Indian Bdellium)

Again a potent herb favouring heart and joint health. The vital component is guggulsterone.

Liquorice (Yashtimadhu)

A soothing herb ideal for comforting irritated membranes and addressing digestive discomfort. Noteworthy constituent: glycyrrhizin.

Turmeric

A golden herb offering anti-inflammatory and antioxidant benefits. The magic ingredient is Curcumin.

Ginger

The digestive system's best mate easing nausea and supporting digestion. Active ingredient: Gingerol.

Boswellia (Indian Frankincense)

An impressive herb offering joint support. The essential component is Boswellic acid.

Gotu Kola (Brahmi)

The brain and nervous system's pal, boosting cognitive function and mental clarity. The constituents mainly include triterpenoid saponins.

Amla (Indian Gooseberry

A potent antioxidant enhancing immune health and promoting longevity. It's rich in Vitamin C.

Amrita (Giloy)

An adaptogen par excellence fostering immunity and vitality. Primary compound: Tinospora Cordifolia.

Bhringraj (False Daisy)

A hair tonic improving hair growth and health. The main component is Wedelolactone.

Kutki (Picrorhiza)

Liver's protector and an effective digestive aid. Key constituents include picroside I and II.

Manjistha (Indian Madder)

A blood purifier addressing skin health. The vital constituent is Munjistin.

Shankhpushpi (Butterfly Pea)

A brain tonic promoting intellect and memory. Principal components include Scopoline and Scopoletin.

Pudina (Mint)

A cooling herb offering digestive relief. Active ingredient: Menthol.

Jatamansi (Spikenard)

An excellent sleep support herb. Important constituents include Jatamansone.

Vasaka (Malabar Nut)

A miraculous herb for the respiratory system. Primary compounds: Vasicine and Vasicinone.

Vidanga (False Black Pepper)

An anti-parasitic herb effective for intestinal health. Active ingredient: Embelin.

Nirgundi (Five-Leaved Chaste Tree)

An analgesic, anti-inflammatory herb for joint health. Relevant constituent: Vitexin.

Punarnava (Boerhavia Diffusa)

A rejuvenate herb catering to kidney and heart health. The important ingredient is Boeravinones.

Bakuchi (Psoralea corylifolia)

A potent herb addressing dermatological conditions. Main constituents: Psoralen.

Guduchi (Heart-Leaved Moonseed)

An adaptogen promoting immunity and reducing stress. Vital constituents: Berberine, giloin, and tinosporol.

Kapoor Kachri (Hedychium spicatum)

A digestive and carminative herb supporting metabolic health. The essential component is Hedycaryol.

This holistic assortment of herbs represents the bedrock of Ayurvedic pharmacy and provide a natural pathway to our well-being journey. It's always advised to use these under proper consultation of Ayurvedic practitioners for optimum benefits and safety.

SOME SPECIFIC CONDITIONS

ARYUVEDA AND MENTAL HEALTH

The Ayurvedic approach to mental health offers a rich tapestry of practices, remedies, and philosophies that have their roots in ancient Indian wisdom. Ayurveda views mental health as an integral part of whole-body wellness, with its perspective adhering to the sagacious correlation between the mind, body, soul, and the universe.

In Ayurveda, the term used for psychology is 'Graha Chikitsa', also referred to as 'Bhut Vidya'. The Ayurvedic approach sees the individual as a unique entity, a dynamic interplay of our bodily constitution, or Prakriti, governed by the three doshas - Vata, Pitta, and Kapha. The doshas are the biophysical forces that orchestrate our physical, mental, emotional, and spiritual health. For mental health, Ayurveda accords significant prominence to the subtle dosha – Vata, specifically Prana Vata, which governs the brain, nerve impulses, and the mind.

Disease, in Ayurvedic terms, is the result of an imbalance. A disturbance in our doshas, mediated by diet, lifestyle choices, or traumatic experiences, disrupts mental harmony. This disruption is responsible for mental disorders like anxiety, depression, attention deficit hyperactivity disorder (ADHD), and even severe conditions like schizophrenia.

Ayurvedic theory places a strong emphasis on preventive care. It encourages cultivating a Sattvic, or pure, lifestyle for maintaining mental equilibrium. Sattvic lifestyle embodies consuming a balanced diet rich in fresh foods, engaging in regular physical activity and meditation, securing ample rest, nurturing positive relationships, and pursuing meaningful activities.

The mind-gut connection is another area where Ayurveda was trailblazing. Ayurveda has always propagated the significance of Agni, the digestive fire and how its suppression leads to Ama, the toxic undigested food particles that harbour disease. Recent research lends weight to the Ayurvedic belief that toxins, or Ama, produced by gut dysbiosis, impact mental health. Therefore, optimizing digestion forms a pivotal pathway in treating many mental health conditions in Ayurveda. Herbs like Ginger, Long Pepper, Black Pepper, and Turmeric serve as beneficial aids in this aspect.

Ayurveda encourages the consumption of brain-nourishing foods like Brahmi (Waterhyssop), Gotu Kola, Ashwagandha, Shankhapushpi (Butterfly Pea), Vacha (Sweet Flag), and Jatamansi (Spikenard), which are revered for their memory-enhancing, antidepressant, anxiolytic, and neuroprotective attributes.

Abhyanga, or Ayurvedic oil massage, is another modality that Ayurveda employs, particularly for Vata-imbalanced disorders. Massages with medicated oils like Sesame, Brahmi, and Bhringraj oil help calm an agitated mind, promote better sleep, and uplift mood.

Powerful therapies like Shirodhara (pouring warm oil on the forehead), Panchakarma (detoxification therapy), and Nasya (nasal administration of medicated oils) have profound healing effects in stress, insomnia, and serious neurodegenerative conditions. The meditative and soothing experience during these therapies enhances the production of happiness hormones like serotonin and dopamine, promoting a sense of tranquillity.

Meditation, Pranayama (breath control practices), and Yoga are the crown jewels of Ayurveda, serving as indispensable tools in managing various mental illnesses. Practices like Trataka (candle gazing), Bhramari (humming bee breath), Nadi Shodhana (alternate nostril breathing), and restorative Yogasana sequences play a pivotal role in grounding the mind, enhancing focus, releasing repressed emotions, combating stress, and fostering mental resilience.

Herbs such as Sarpagandha (Serpentina root), which contain the powerful alkaloid Reserpine, have been traditionally used in Ayurveda for their calming properties. Modern pharmacology also uses this compound in the treatment of hypertension, anxiety, and certain psychotic disorders.

Unlike the reductionist view of modern medicine, which aims at symptom suppression, Ayurveda's holistic and personalized approach aims at the root cause - balancing doshas, restoring digestion, rejuvenating nervous system function, and promoting mental serenity. Ayurveda respects individual uniqueness, and its treatments are tailored to the person's unique constitution, offering a rounded, side-effect-free solution for mental health disorders. It's a testament to the timeless relevance of this ancient wisdom in our current era marked by frequent mental health challenges.

The safe harbouring thought in the heart of Ayurveda is the conviction that mental health, akin to a calm, clear lake mirroring the cosmos, is our natural state, achievable through the mindful regulation of our lifestyle, diet, thoughts, and actions.

Embracing Ayurveda empowers us to be the proud curators of our mind-body health rather than feeling like bewildered victims of our minds. With an open mind, and under the guidance of professional Ayurvedic practitioners, anyone suffering from a mental health condition can tread the soothing path of Ayurvedic healing and experience the transformation unfolding in its own time, nurturing their journey from fear and distress to peace and well-being.

ARYUVEDA AND RHEUMATIC CONDITIONS

In the ancient science of Ayurveda, the deep-reaching influence of this healing tradition provides a comprehensive approach to rheumatic disorders, focused on holistic healing rather than symptom management.

In Ayurveda, a rheumatic disorder, termed 'Amavata', is fundamentally governed by Ama, the toxic byproducts of inefficient digestion. Ama, paired with provoked Vata dosha, is carried to different parts of the body, including the joints. It results in symptoms like joint pain, inflammation, stiffness, fever, and general weakness. These are remarkably similar to symptoms seen in modern-day rheumatic diseases such as rheumatoid arthritis, osteoarthritis, lupus, and gout.

To counteract rheumatic disorders, Ayurveda employs a multi-pronged strategy: dietary adjustments, lifestyle modifications, herbal remedies, Panchakarma (detoxification procedure), and Yoga.

Diet lies at the heart of Ayurvedic therapy. Consuming warm, light, and easily digestible foods boosts the digestive fire, Agni, preventing Ama formation. Green leafy vegetables, pumpkin, bitter gourd, bottle gourd, carrot, garlic, fenugreek, coriander, turmeric, ginger, black pepper, and cumin are beneficial for their anti-inflammatory properties.

Sounds like a delicious warming soup to me!

Conversely, it is advisable to avoid cold, heavy, and hard-to-digest foods, including processed items, cold drinks, and nightshade vegetables like tomatoes, white potatoes, peppers, and eggplants, as they can aggravate symptoms.

Movement is medicine! Gentle and regular exercise, particularly Yoga, is advised to enhance circulation and flexibility. Yoga asanas such as Sukhasana (Easy Pose), Viparita Karani (Legs Up The Wall Pose), Setu Band Sarvangasana (Bridge Pose), and Shishosana (Puppy Pose) are beneficial.

Ayurvedic herbal remedies have a significant role in rheumatic disorders. Their administration is typically under the guidance of an experienced Ayurvedic practitioner. Some of the potent Ayurvedic herbs for rheumatic disorders include Guggulu, Ashwagandha, Triphala, Dashamoola, Shallaki, and Nirgundi.

Decoction of Dashamoola, a group of ten beneficial herbs, is excellent for reducing inflammation and pain. Shallaki or Indian Frankincense, has been extensively studied for its potent anti-inflammatory and pain-relieving properties. Simultaneously, Guggulu, particularly in the form of Yograj Guggulu or Kaishore Guggulu, can be beneficial for rheumatic disorders as a potent anti-inflammatory and immune-modulating herb. Ashwagandha, often hailed as Indian ginseng, is notable for its immune-balancing and stress-relieving properties.

Panchakarma, the Ayurvedic detoxification procedure, particularly in the form of Virechana (therapeutic purgation) and Basti (therapeutic enema), can be beneficial when performed under expert supervision. Panchakarma procedures aid in eliminating Ama, calming aggravated Vata, and reducing inflammation, leading to relief from symptoms.

Ayurvedic treatment for rheumatic disorders also emphasizes lifestyle modifications to support the healing process and prevent disease exacerbation. Patients should ensure they have regular sleep patterns, manage their stress levels, and avoid exposure to cold and damp environments.

Please remember that Ayurvedic treatment is highly personalized, taking into consideration the individual's constitution, severity and nature of the disease, age, and overall health. Always consult with an experienced Ayurvedic practitioner who can guide you through the healing journey.

Adopting Ayurveda's principles will not only address the root-cause of rheumatic disorders but will also guide you towards wholesome well-being. Treatment can sometimes be a lengthy process, requiring patience, trust, and commitment. Be consistent, take one step at a time, and trust the wisdom of this age-old science. Above all, remember that healing happens when you are an active participant. Through Ayurveda, you reclaim your health, allowing your body and mind to return to their natural state of balance. Good health then becomes not just an end goal, but an enjoyable daily journey.

You don't have to fight rheumatic disorders alone. Let Ayurveda, with its holistic wisdom, shine the light on your path towards vitality and vibrant health.

ARYUVEDA AND ARTHRITIC CONDITIONS

The grandeur of Ayurveda lies in its holistic approach to health and its capacity to tackle disease at its root instead of just symptomatic treatment. Arthritis, known as 'Sandhivata' in Ayurvedic terms, is a condition it can manage successfully.

Referring to inflammation of the joints, arthritis is notorious for resulting in symptoms like joint pain, stiffness, and decreased range of motion. Its chief forms include osteoarthritis, rheumatoid arthritis, and gout. In Ayurveda, arthritis is perceived as Vata dosha's aggravated condition, especially affecting the joints. Various factors like improper diet, sedentary lifestyle, ageing, and climatic conditions can be responsible for this imbalance.

To appease the symptoms of arthritis, Ayurveda recommends a four-pronged approach: Ideal diet, Lifestyle modifications, Herbal remedies, and Panchakarma.

A balanced and nutritious diet sits at the core of Ayurvedic arthritis treatment. Warm, light, and easy-to-digest foods that balance Vata are recommended to prevent Ama accumulation. Barley, Moong dal, Garlic, Turmeric, Asafoetida, Drumstick, and Bitter gourd are particularly conducive to arthritis management because of their anti-inflammatory qualities.

In contrast, avoid cold, heavy, and hard-to-digest foods which can lead to Ama formation and Vata aggravation. Processed foods, bread-filled items, cold drinks, and nightshade vegetables can serve to exasperate symptoms.

A sedentary lifestyle can significantly increase arthritic difficulties. Mild exercises, preferably under the rising sun, can help to improve circulation and reduce stiffness. Yoga poses such as Trikonasana (Triangle Pose), Marjariasana (Cat Pose), Setu Bandhasana (Bridge Pose), and gentle Sun Salutation sequences can improve joint mobility and flexibility.

The repertoire of Ayurvedic herbs is potent for coping with arthritic conditions. Ashwagandha, Guggulu, Turmeric, Ginger, and Boswellia are powerful herbs used in managing arthritis. Guggulu (Commiphora mukul) exhibits potent anti-inflammatory and analgesic properties. Shallaki or Boswellia Serrata also shows remarkable inflammation-controlling complexity, along with protective effects on the cartilage.

Panchakarma, Ayurveda's reputed detoxification process, forms an integral part of comprehensive arthritis treatment. Procedures, especially Bashpa Sweda (Steam Therapy) and Abhyanga (Oil Massage), can vastly improve joint mobility and reduce pain. Virechana (Purgation) and Basti (Enema) can be beneficial in severe conditions, where a significant accumulation of toxins has occurred.

Lifestyle holds an important place in managing arthritis. Practice regular sleeping habits and beneficial therapeutic practices such as warm oil massages. Avoid exposure to cold and damp environments, as these may increase Vata, aggravating joint pain and stiffness.

Remember to always consult an experienced Ayurvedic healthcare professional for personalized guidance. While these treatments can offer noticeable relief, they do require patience, as eliminating accumulated toxins and restoring balance to the body's systems, takes time.

In essence, Ayurveda does more than mere symptom management of arthritic diseases. It aims to restore balance, addressing the root cause, and through this, brings about lasting relief. Certainly, managing arthritic conditions successfully is a reality within the wisdom of Ayurveda. Combining Ayurvedic directives on diet, lifestyle, herbal remedies, and therapies under proper guidance, can work wonders.

Finally, patients should not view arthritis as an isolated ailment affecting their joints but instead understand that it is intricately linked to overall health and wellness. Ayurveda encourages becoming partners in one's own healing journey, by making wise dining choices, living an active lifestyle, and managing stress effectively.

In the grand play of life, you're not merely an actor but a director of your health and well-being too. Lead your life's play charmingly with Ayurveda's wisdom, considering arthritis not as a life sentence, but a sign from within that your body needs vital attention and care. Allow Ayurveda to bring you from stiffness and pain to fluidity and freedom.

ARYUVEDA AND ECZEMA

Resorting to the 5000-year-old wisdom of Ayurveda to address eczema, pronounced as 'Vicharchika', holds considerable promise. Translating literally as 'that which spreads', eczema epitomizes an aggravated state of Pitta dosha, where the fire element in the skin is disturbed, disrupting the normal functioning of the skin's protective barrier. This manifests in dryness, inflammation, and itching.

To manage eczema successfully, Ayurveda presents an all-encompassing strategy: the right Ayurvedic diet, lifestyle modifications, potent herbals, and Panchakarma.

Diet being the essential life force, Ayurveda assigns it a pivotal role to maintain and restore health. Opt for 'cooling' foods that pacify Pitta, like cucumbers, ripe bananas, green beans, zucchini, winter squash, and leafy greens. Being rich in water, these foods keep the body hydrated and skin nourished. Avoid hot, spicy, oily, and processed foods that aggravate Pitta and can stimulate skin inflammation.

The adoption of a healthy lifestyle reinforces the effect of a balanced diet. Maintain a regular sleep pattern and practice yoga and meditation to manage stress, a common eczema trigger. Asanas like Sheetali pranayama (Cooling Breath), Chandrabhedi pranayama (Left Nostril Breathing), and Shavasana (Corpse Pose) are beneficial.

Ayurvedic herbs form another powerful tool to keep eczema at bay. Herbs like Neem, Turmeric, Aloe Vera, Sandalwood, and Jasmine are particularly favored. Neem, an excellent detoxifier and blood purifier, can help eliminate the toxins causing eczema. Aloe Vera's cooling properties soothe the skin, reducing inflammation, and itching. Drinkable Aloe Vera juice can also be used for its purifying properties.

Applying a mixture of Sandalwood powder with rose water can calm the skin due to its cooling effect. Jasmine flowers used in oils and creams can help improve the skin condition. Internally, Ayurvedic formulations like Kaishore Guggulu, Arogyavardhini Vati, and Mahatiktaka Ghrita can be fruitful.

Panchakarma, with its various specialized therapies, forms a significant part of Ayurvedic eczema treatment. Two special therapies—Virechana (therapeutic purgation) and Takradhara (streaming buttermilk on the forehead)—are used. These assist in eliminating the toxins from the body and balancing Pitta dosha.

Remember, no two eczema cases are alike. Always consult an Ayurvedic practitioner who can offer a nuanced understanding of your specific condition and devise a personalized treatment plan. Achieving a complete cure for this chronic condition might require a continuous and systematic approach.

Ayurveda's steady approach ensures the complete reversal of eczema, moulding an amicable relationship between you and your skin. It empowers you to become an active participant in your healing process rather than being a passive recipient of treatment.

Eczema, though chronically uncomfortable, could be a useful signal too. It nudges you to look beneath the skin surface and introspect your 'ha-bitual' habits. Ayurveda doesn't merely strive to soothe eczema's symptoms; it aims to eradicate its root causes, guiding you towards conscious living and a healthy skin-friendly lifestyle.

In essence, acknowledging Ayurveda's principles allows you not only to put a robust fight against eczema but also to redefine your skin relationship holistically. You won't just combat the outer 'itch', but also take care of the inner 'itch' for a deeper connection with your skin.

Eczema, together with Ayurveda, could be your stepping stone towards illuminating the hidden aspects of your existence you might have otherwise missed. So, brace yourself for the journey, and who knows, you might fall in love with your skin all over again!

ARYUVEDA AND PSORIASIS

Diving into the profound essence of Ayurveda presents an effective solution to managing psoriasis, regarded as 'Kitibha' or 'Ekakushta' in Ayurvedic terminology. Specifically attributed to the discordance and overactivity of the Vata and Kapha doshas, psoriasis manifests itself as a chronic skin disorder marked by flaky, silvery scales, inflammation, and dryness on the skin.

In its pursuit to heal psoriasis from the root cause, Ayurveda prescribes a multi-faceted approach: optimal dietary practices, life-affirming behavioural routines, an array of natural herbs, and Panchkarma.

In dietary practices, Ayurveda acknowledges the profound interconnection between the gut and skin. It therefore recommends Vata and Kapha pacifying foods that are warm, light, and easy to digest. This would include a generous incorporation of fresh fruits and vegetables, whole grains, seeds, and legumes. Allium vegetables like garlic, onions, and leeks, rich in naturally occurring sulfur, could enhance the skin's health and appearance.

Stay away from energy-draining and gut-compromising foods like processed goods, canned items, excess salt, spicy foods, and refined sugars. Dairy products, red meat, citrus fruits, gluten, and nightshade vegetables like tomatoes, potatoes, bell peppers, and eggplants may exacerbate the condition in some individuals, and it is best to limit these.

Ayurveda also underlines the importance of comprehensive lifestyle changes to counteract psoriasis effectively. Cultivate a routine, embracing yoga and meditation to keep stress - a common psoriasis trigger - at bay. Specific asanas like Tadasana (Palm Tree Pose), Shishuasana (Child Pose), and Vajrasana (Diamond Pose) could be practiced. Embrace a Sun salutation sequence, invigorating the skin cells.

Herbs hold a special place in Ayurvedic therapeutics for psoriasis. Neem, aloe vera, turmeric, and guggul are particularly effective. Neem, a powerful blood purifier and immune booster, can be used both topically and internally. Aloe Vera, due to its moisturizing and healing properties, can soothe psoriatic skin, reduce inflammation and scaling. Turmeric, potent in antioxidant and anti-inflammatory properties, could be beneficial both orally and topically. Guggul, a traditional Ayurvedic herb, is known to reduce the redness, thickness, and scaling of psoriatic skin.

Finally, Panchkarma, the crown jewel of Ayurveda, offers systemic cleansing and detoxification to purify the body off waste material known as Ama, piled up in the body. Treatments like Vamana (therapeutic vomiting) and Virechana (therapeutic purgation) are used to cleanse the body and restore balance.

However, it is critical to bear in mind that because psoriasis is a complex and individualistic disease, every person's experience will differ significantly. It is therefore highly recommended to seek personalized advice from an experienced Ayurvedic practitioner, providing a careful diagnosis and a customized treatment plan.

By harnessing Ayurveda's wisdom, you could triumph over the grip of psoriasis. Its integrative approach aims to promote balanced living, and in doing so, creates a space for your skin to introspect, self-repair and rejuvenate.

Psoriasis, often a cause of despair, could paradoxically elevate you, heralding a journey towards your innate health. Ayurveda allows you to transform that despair into a window to understand your body better. It serves as a reminder to revisit life choices, consume consciously, live mindfully, and embrace a deeper kinship with nature.

Indeed, with Ayurveda, you grow beyond being merely a silent spectator of the disease. You become an active participant, an 'artist' who perfectly moulds the 'clay' of your body. It urges you to rise above considering psoriasis as just a skin disorder, recognizing it as an opportunity for internal self-discovery and external skin transformation.

With its roots in natural wisdom, Ayurveda arms you with self-care tools that empower you to embark on a skin healing journey. In this journey, you might not merely vanquish psoriasis but discover a newer 'you' - radiant and unfettered. After all, your skin is a testimony to your life's narrative; let it not be a tale of encumbrance but a story of skin renewal and celebration.

ARYUVEDA AND ASTHMA

Peering through the lens of the timeless and holistic medical system of Ayurveda provides a unique perspective on managing asthma, or 'Tamaka Swasa' as referred to in Ayurvedic literature. This chronic respiratory disorder signifies the aggravation of Kapha dosha in the stomach, which later emerges in the chest area causing blockage in the airflow.

Ayurveda strives to manage asthma not merely as a lung disorder, but as a repercussion of overall physiological imbalance. It underlines a comprehensive approach that includes specially curated Ayurvedic diet, incorporation of suitable lifestyle routines, usage of beneficial herbs, and application of Panchakarma therapies.

First and foremost, it's pivotal to address diet, the foundation stone of Ayurvedic healing. Foods that boost your immunity while balancing the Kapha dosha help the body resist asthma. Foods like carrots, radishes, honey, lean meats such as chicken and turkey, and spices like turmeric, black pepper, and ginger can be potent for asthmatic patients. Hydrating the body with warm fluids or herbal teas can help keep lung passages moist and aid in removing toxins.

Ayurveda suggests refraining from heavy, fried, processed, and dairy foods, which can increase Kapha and create Ama (toxins) leading to increased phlegm production. Alcohol, smoking and high consumption of caffeine are also discouraged for they aggravate Vata and Pitta, and can tamper respiratory functioning.

On the lifestyle front, it's crucial to harmonize the mind, body, and soul to manage asthma effectively. Breathing exercises or Pranayama, such as Anulom Vilom (alternate nostril breathing) can help in clearing the airways for smooth breathing. Regular practice of yoga could be beneficial to struggling lungs as asanas like Bhujangasana, Ardha Matsyendrasana, Pavanamuktasana enhance the lung capacity, increase oxygen supply and help pacify and balance the aggravated doshas.

Herbal formulations hold the key as they impart strength to the lungs and can help manage asthma symptoms. Herbs like Tulsi (Holy basil), Vasaka, Licorice, and Piper longum are preferred. Tulsi offers relief from congestion and can enhance immunity. Vasaka, a popular herb for respiratory disorders, calms the respiratory tract. Liquorice's anti-inflammatory properties soothe the lungs. Piper longum, beneficial for respiratory function, aids in removing congestion and promoting easy breathing.

Further, the power of Ayurveda's deep cleansing and detoxification therapy, Panchakarma, cannot be emphasized enough. Nasya (nasal insufflation) can be effective against chest congestion. Vamana (therapeutic vomiting) can be beneficial for expulsion of excess Kapha dosha.

However, remember that every individual has a unique Dosha makeup, and the mentioned treatments may differ in terms of effectiveness. Hence, it becomes essential to consult a certified Ayurvedic practitioner for a custom-made treatment plan catering to individual needs.

Thus, with Ayurveda, a healthier you is not a far-fetched aspiration but a daily reality. As well as remedying the immediate discomfort of asthma, it unearths the underlying causes and induces positive transformations in dietary habits and lifestyle. It enlightens us that we are not victims of an irreversible disease; we are robust entities capable of self-healing and restoration.

Asthma, often seen as an adversary, could be an ally in understanding the nuances of your body better. The disease could pave the path towards an agreeable and cohesive system of well-being, while Ayurveda could guide you towards discarding life-threatening habits and fostering healthier substitutes.

In a nutshell, Ayurveda's role doesn't cease at treating asthma; it guides you towards a balanced state of vitality where you stand strong, not despite asthma, but because of it. With Ayurveda, it's not just about healing asthma; it's about healing the self, being one's own health's architect, and breathing free, now and always.

ARYUVEDA AND ADHT

Attention Deficit Hyperactivity Disorder (ADHD), identified in Ayurveda as 'Unmada', is primarily due to an imbalance in the Vata dosha. This neurological disorder, characterized by an unwarranted propensity for inattention, hyperactivity, and impulsivity, holds the potential to impair an individual's daily functioning gravely.

Ayurveda, with its extensive understanding of the individual's constitution (Prakriti) and the intricacies of the three Doshas - Vata, Pitta, and Kapha, offers insightful strategies for managing ADHD. The intervention primarily revolves around behavioural modifications, dietary changes, Ayurvedic therapies, yoga, and the utilization of medicinal herbs, offering a holistic treatment paradigm.

Ayurveda proposes dietary modifications as a vital element of the ADHD management strategy. Consuming Vata balancing foods that are fresh, warm, juicy, and easily digestible, can be truly beneficial. This can include foods high in protein and complex carbohydrates, calming herbal teas, fresh fruits and vegetables, dairy products like milk and ghee, nuts, and seeds.

Ayurveda advises against intake of raw, cold, and dry foods, excessive sweet, bitter or astringent foods, processed foods laden with artificial additives and highly caffeinated drinks. Such food items are believed to aggravate the Vata Dosha and subsequently increase symptoms of ADHD.

The lifestyle that one leads plays a significant part in influencing the course of ADHD. Ayurveda suggests regular adherence to a sleep schedule, routine exercise, spending time outdoors in nature and abiding by a structured daily routine. Nasnasya therapy, the nasal administration of medicated oils or ghee is particularly beneficial in managing the symptoms.

The practice of yoga and meditation can induce profound positive changes in managing ADHD symptoms. Yoga asanas that encourage balance and coordination are particularly beneficial. Pranayama practices such as Nadi Shodhana (alternate nostril breathing) can also be incorporated to calm the mind and balance the Doshas. The practice of Transcendental Meditation (TM), in particular, has shown promising results in improving attention span and curbing impulsive behaviour in children with ADHD.

Ayurveda enumerates several herbs that play an influential role in managing ADHD symptoms. Few among them are Brahmi (Bacopa monnieri), Mandukaparni (Centella asiatica), and Vacha (Acorus calamus), all well-known for their mind-calming properties. Ashwagandha (Withania somnifera), a well-documented adaptogenic herb, assists in stress reduction and in enhancing concentration levels. Regular consumption of these herbs, under the guidance of an experienced Ayurvedic practitioner, can be immensely helpful.

Panchakarma (five actions) therapies can play an essential role in eliminating toxins, which are known to interfere with cognitive functions. These purification therapies aim to balance the doshas and ensure they are functioning optimally. Abhyanga (Ayurveda body massage) and Shirodhara (pouring of warm oil on forehead) can be extremely calming, pacifying the Vata dosha and helping improve attention span.

It's important to note, however, the effectiveness and appropriateness of these interventions can vary substantially from person to person, considering our unique constitutions. It is, therefore, highly recommended that those diagnosed with ADHD consult an experienced Ayurvedic practitioner for personalized guidance.

Approaching ADHD through the holistic perspective of Ayurveda provides more than just symptom management. It encourages a comprehensive lifestyle change that promotes overall health, wellness, and balance. Ayurveda endows the enduring sentiment of wholesome living, and an understanding of the innate nature of ADHD, unveiling the potential to transform this neurological disorder into a stepping stone towards self-discovery and growth.

Redefining ADHD as a functional diversity rather than a disability, Ayurveda reassures that with the right therapeutic strategy and lifestyle changes, living with ADHD can possibly transmute from chronic struggle to an acquired skill of managing energies. In achieving this, Ayurveda goes past adjusting the ADHD aspect of a person it aids in nurturing a well-rounded, balanced individual who is not just surviving with ADHD but flourishing amidst it.

ARYUVEDA AND OPCD

Obsessive-Compulsive Personality Disorder (OCPD), a pervasive condition characterized by a chronic preoccupation with rules, orderliness, and control, could create significant distress and disability. As a multifaceted holistic system, Ayurveda offers a unique approach to OCPD treatment.

The Ayurvedic alternative concept views the mind and body as a single entity where mental unrest has direct physical implications. OCPD in Ayurveda could be primarily attributed to imbalances in Vata Dosha, responsible for functions related to movement, thinking, and nervous system regulation.

Through comprehensive lifestyle changes, medicinal herbs, Panchakarma therapies, meditation practices, and dietary adjustments, Ayurveda provides a holistic solution for managing OCPD and its symptoms.

Let's begin with the essence of OCPD management – diet. As per Ayurveda, dietary rules (Pathya) play a vital role. Ayurveda advocates a 'Sattvic' diet, which intrinsically means food that escalates purity, knowledge, and harmony. Sattvic foods foster clarity and perception, pacify the mind, and help promote tranquillity and creativity, making it easier to let go of control-oriented tendencies. Some examples of Sattvic food include dairy products, nuts, seeds, ripe fruits, legumes, and fresh vegetables. Consuming these foods assist in balancing Vata Dosha and pacifying the mind.

Next, Ayurveda pays paramount attention to 'Dincharya' or daily routine. Establishing a set daily routine helps to balance the Vata dosha—the consistency and predictability of a daily routine feed into the OCPD's need for control, offering a healthy outlet for it. Regularly waking up, eating, working, exercising, and sleeping at the same times can be incredibly stabilizing and calming, providing grounding and soothing the nervous system.

Sleep is another crucial factor. Ayurveda encourages good sleep hygiene to support mental wellbeing. In OCPD, where the mind tends to be overactive with recurrent, persistent thoughts, it can sometimes lead to sleep disturbances. Hence, paying heed to maintaining proper sleep schedule and quality is incredibly significant.

Physical activity is also an important component. Ayurveda suggests that regular exercise, especially yoga, can be an effective tool for managing OCPD. It not only helps balance the doshas but also aids in relieving stress and enabling better focus. Specific 'asanas' or yoga poses can help to mitigate the effects of OCPD. For instance, Balasana (Child's Pose) eases the mind and provides a sense of calm from excessive perfectionism and controlling tendencies.

Moreover, Ayurveda offers numerous herbs with profound healing properties. Bacopa Monnieri (Brahmi), Centella Asiatica (Gotu Kola), and Withania Somnifera (Ashwagandha) among others, are recognized for their anxiety-reducing and mind-calming effects. Under the guidance of a proficient Ayurvedic practitioner, administration of these herbs can significantly aid in managing OCPD symptoms.

'Panchakarma', the purification and detoxification therapy, is another potent remedy. These therapies assist in purging toxins, promoting physiological strength and stability, eventually leading to a balanced state of mind.

The power of mindful meditation and breathing exercises, also known as 'Pranayama,' is another instrumental tool. By encouraging 'present moment' orientation, meditation helps to break away from the clutches of obsessive thoughts and offers a sense of control.

That said, all symptoms and individuals are unique. Therefore, any Ayurvedic intervention should be carried out under the expert supervision of a trained Ayurvedic practitioner to ensure safety and efficacy.

In the wake of chronic conditions like OCPD, the teachings of Ayurveda can bring solace to troubled minds. The Ayurvedic approach equips you with tools to lead the mind into serenity and balance, transforming mental health challenges into an intimate journey of self-understanding and healing, connecting the dots between mind, body, spirit, and the universe.

Through its utterly holistic approach to health and wellness, Ayurveda teaches how to beautifully build a life, instead of just spending a lifetime. It teaches us that the right balance in life is attainable and sustainable, one just needs guidance and consistent practice. The reality of OCPD, through the perspective of Ayurveda, becomes bearable, and dare say, conquerable.

ARYUVEDA AND COPD

Chronic Obstructive Pulmonary Disease (COPD) is a prevalent, persistent lung disease typified by breathlessness and diminished respiratory function. Strikingly, Ayurveda, with its rich ancient knowledge, can provide supplementary management strategies aimed at enhancing the quality of life for those living with COPD.

Ayurveda addresses COPD through a multidimensional approach, combining specialized dietary measures, specific exercises, herbal remedies, lifestyle modifications, and cleansing therapies to manage the symptoms and slow disease progression.

In Ayurveda, COPD is called 'Tamaksvasa', considered primarily a 'Kapha' dosha disorder but with significant involvement of 'Vata' and 'Pitta' doshas too. However, the treatments may vary based on the predominance of Doshas involved in the disease pathogenesis.

Diet plays a cardinal role in managing COPD from an Ayurvedic perspective. Consuming a prana-rich diet, abundant in life force and vitality, can be highly beneficial. Foods high in prana include fresh fruits, vegetables, whole grains, nuts, seeds, and legumes. They not only strengthen the immune system but also help clear the airways and control inflammation, attributing to COPD.

Agni (digestive fire) is given profound importance in Ayurveda. A healthy agni results in good digestion, assimilation and strong immunity. In COPD, balancing the digestion can be essential in suppressing further production of Ama (toxic byproduct of improper digestion), which fuels further inflammation.

Ayurveda acknowledges that COPD sufferers can face difficulties with physical activity due to breathlessness. However, mild exercises like Pranayama (breathing exercises), Yoga, and walking are encouraged. Pranayama and gentle yoga asanas can help strengthen respiratory muscles, enhance lung capacity, and improve oxygen saturation in the blood.

Next, the use of beneficial herbs plays an essential part in Ayurveda. Herbs like Liquorice, Guggulu, Tulsi, and Vasaka have a formidable reputation for their broncho dilatory, anti-inflammatory, and antioxidant properties. Proper utilization of such medicinal herbs, under supervision, can improve respiratory strength, reduce phlegm production, and fight bronchial inflammation.

Ayurveda strongly believes in the control of stress as a supportive measure for COPD management. Stress and anxiety can cause exacerbations- worsen shortness of breath, and trigger COPD flare-ups. Strategies like meditation and mindfulness can help improve overall quality of life, reduce stress, and increase coping skills for dealing with the disease.

Another pivotal treatment in Ayurveda is Panchakarma- a five-step body purification and rejuvenation process. Within Panchakarma, therapies like Vamana (controlled emesis), Nasya (nasal medication instillation) and Virechana (purgation) are employed to detoxify the body, remove excessive Kapha, improve digestion, and boost immunity.

Moreover, various Ayurvedic rejuvenating or 'Rasayana' therapies are recommended to boost lung health and immunity. Chyawanprash, a herbal jam made from an amalgamation of health-enhancing herbs, is renowned for its rejuvenating and immune-boosting properties, proving beneficial in managing COPD.

Finally, proper sleep and rest are deemed essential in Ayurveda. It insists on maintaining a regular sleep schedule for healing and restoring energy.

Even though Ayurveda offers substantial methods to manage COPD, it's not a substitute for mainstream COPD treatment. It's a complementary approach, and any attempts to follow such regimens should be under the careful supervision of healthcare professionals and Ayurvedic practitioners with appropriate knowledge and experience in dealing with COPD.

Therefore, with its unique holistic approach, Ayurveda leads the way, offering both symptomatic and complementary interventions for COPD. Ayurveda not only focuses on the bodily ailment but also the socio-spiritual aspects, paving the way for comprehensive health and well-being. Amidst the distress caused by COPD, the Ayurvedic approach brings hope, resilience, and a new perspective to life.

SOME GENTLE EXERCISES FOR EVERYONE

Ayurveda, the ancient Indian healing science, offers a holistic roadmap of wellness encompassing diet, lifestyle, herbs, and not forgetting – exercise. Exercise enhances circulation, zest, and longevity, cleanses toxins, nurtures the body, and anchors our consciousness in the here and now. Remember, the ultimate aim is balancing our body's constitutions, or Doshas – Vata, Pitta, and Kapha.

For beginners embarking on the Ayurvedic journey, the synergy of Ayurveda and Yoga offers an ideal entrance to physical wellness. Gentle yoga poses, stretches, and breathing exercises create an intricate symphony that harmonizes the body's energies with the mind's waves.

Before we start, a crucial principle of Ayurveda to remember is exerting to half of your capacity. You should feel recharged, not drained, after these exercises.

Tadasana (Mountain Pose)

Stand tall and relaxed. Distribute weight evenly across your feet. Breathe smoothly and visualize yourself as a sturdy mountain.

2. Balasana (Child's Pose)

Kneel on a mat. Relax your buttocks onto your heels, stretch your hands forward, and rest your forehead gently on the mat. Breathing deeply in this pose helps unwind the mind and rejuvenates your energy.

3. Anjaneyasana (Low Lunge)

Step back into a runner's lunge. Lower your back knee and relax the top of your foot on the floor. Press your hands on your front knee and extend your chest. This pose is excellent for hip flexibility and strength.

Viparita Karani (Legs-Up-The-Wall Poses)

Lie down near a wall and elevate your legs against it. Extend your arms comfortably by your sides. This pose is fantastic for quieting the mind and promoting relaxation.

Sukhasana (Easy Pose)

Cross your legs comfortably, rest your hands on your knees, elongate your spine, and breathe deeply. This pose is excellent for grounding and centering our energies.

Ardha Matsyendrasana (Half Lord of the Fishes Pose)

In a seated position, bend your right knee and place your foot past the left knee. Hold your right knee with your left arm while twisting your upper body to the right. This pose is good for spinal flexibility and abdominal organs.

Savasana (Corpse Pose)

Lay flat on your back, legs comfortably apart, hands by your sides, palms facing up. Doing absolutely nothing in this pose is paradoxically 'everything'. Savasana helps digest the physical and mental benefits of the practice.

Breathing Exercises (Pranayama) are potent tools to fortify lung capacity, soothe the nervous system, and cultivate clarity and calm.

Diaphragmatic breathing

Place your hand on your abdomen, relaxing your shoulders and chest. Inhale deeply so that your hand rises. Exhale, allowing your hand to descend. This slow, deep breathing aids in calming the anxious mind.

Nadi Shodhana (Alternate Nostril Breathing)

Press your thumb on the right nostril, inhale through the left nostril, then press the ring finger on the left nostril, and exhale through the right nostril. Repeat the process starting with an inhale on the right side. This balancing breath cultivates mental tranquillity and clarity.

Brahmarī Prānāyāma (Buzzing Bee Breath)

Close your eyes, plug your ears with your fingers and take a deep breath in. On exhale, make a slow, smooth buzzing sound like a bee. This practice calms the mind and nurtures the throat.

Kapalabhati (Skull Shining Breath)

Sit comfortably, take a gentle breath in, and release a sharp exhale from your lower belly, sucking it in. Let the inhale happen passively. Kapalabhati is an energizing breath that cleanses the lungs and mind.

Ayurveda also advocates self-massage (Abhyanga) with warm, dosha-specific oils before bath, a gentle form of exercise that nourishes the skin, muscles, and nerves. In addition, a peaceful walk in nature or an easy-paced bicycle ride also perfectly aligns with the Ayurvedic principles of gentle movement, soaking in the healing energy of Mother Nature.

Remember, Ayurveda emphasizes the unique needs of each individual. It's never one-size-fits-all. For Vata constitutions, calming exercises accompanied with ample rest is preferable. Pitta individuals can benefit from moderate, enjoyable exercises in cooler environments, to prevent over-heating. Vigorous action suits Kapha personas best, but starting slowly and gradually is key.

Consistency, rather than intensity, is the golden rule of adopting these exercises in your daily routine. Pay attention to your body's language and modify as required. Over time, they will become effortless, almost second nature, strengthening the body, enlivening the spirits, and weaving their way into a harmonious Ayurvedic lifestyle.

Remember, your Ayurvedic journey is a marathon, not a sprint. It's a slow, steady, and loving commitment to yourself and your well-being. The ultimate goal is not 'perfection,' but the ongoing journey of learning, growth, and profound self-discovery. So, lace your journey with love, compassion, and patience, and watch your life transform like magic.

PERSONALIZATION IN MARKETING

A CUTTING-EDGE, STEP-BY-STEP GUIDE TO ACQUIRE USEFUL SKILLS, GROW YOUR COMPANY TO MILLIONS DOLLARS, AND PROVIDE CUSTOMIZED EXPERIENCES FOR YOUR CLIENTS

RICHARD N. WILLIAMS

TABLE OF CONTENTS